Dying To Be Thin

A Journey Through Weight-Loss Surgery
(Exposing the Risks of the Gastric-Bypass Procedure)

By Stephanie French

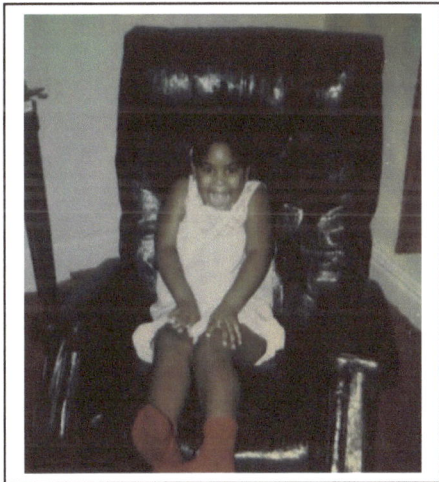

Copyright 2006

Dying To Be Thin
By Stephanie French

Copyright 2006 by Stephanie French
Note: This book is not a substitute for seeking professional help at a time when one is contemplating diets, surgery or weight-reduction mechanisms.

Published by
M.O.R.E. Publishers Corp.
P.O. Box 38285
St. Louis, MO 63138
(314) 383-7410   MOREPublishersCO@aol.com
Angelee Coleman Grider, editor and founder

Cover photo release permission by Glamour Shots of St. Louis.

Cover Design by Edwin Marcellus T. Grider

Published in the United States
ISBN: 978-0-9719984-7-6

SFrench32@Yahoo.com

Stephanie French

DEDICATION

I dedicate this book to Mrs. Freda Kane who dared to follow through on her dreams.

If the deceased could talk, she probably would say….

"I died trying to become thin/Not realizing beauty comes from within/On a quest to become what some thought I should be/Forgetting God had a unique plan for me/Now I am dead and my breath has ceased/Remember to love yourself for who you are/God made you a special shining star." Greta Long, like many other individuals, paid the ultimate price in her quest to become thin: her life.

Dying to be Thin is a must-read book for anyone contemplating gastric-bypass surgery as it reveals a side of this procedure that few dare talk about. This book also challenges traditional views about beauty and shows its readers that our true value comes, not from conforming to what others think we should be, but from discovering who God made us to be.

Preface

This book is my testimony about how good God is to me. Even during my disobedience of wanting to have weight-loss surgery, He still blessed the work of my hands. Believe me that if you trust in God, and let Him lead, you will finally realize that anything is possible.

Amen

About the Author

Stephanie French was born and reared in Amory, Mississippi. She now resides in St. Louis, Missouri.

She has three children named Demario, Ashley and Amber.

Stephanie French is a licensed youth minister and founder of "PROJECT SELF", a self-esteem program for young women.

Dying
To Be
Thin

Inside

Introduction
Finding a Dying Friend
(The voice of Greta Long, the one who died)

Stephanie and I met on a cold, November morning as we both sat in that dark, gloomy doctor's office – both crumpled over in pain. As we began to talk we realized that we were both having some of the same postoperative complications due to weight loss surgery:
1. severe constipation
2. vomiting
3. dehydration
4. abdominal excruciating pain

"I'm hurting! The nurse called Stephanie's name first," Greta managed to say to her sister Mary, sitting next to her.

"She said she wasn't hurting too badly to keep her from walking," Greta thought to herself.

"I am grateful that Mary came from Atlanta to take care of me."

Stephanie and I said our good-byes. I was still sitting next to my sister and Lavenus, Stephanie's friend stayed quietly seated.

"I'm drifting off. Maybe that's a good thing. I won't keep feeling the pain".

Just briefly Greta began reminiscing about her initial choice to have the surgery.

1

"Oh, no!" I suddenly screamed. A sharp pin-piercing pain shot through my body. "I see that every choice has consequences, and my decision seem to be having a negative effect on me, my family and my friends."

"Why is everything so different now?"

"I am always in pain!"

"Yesterday was even worst than this pain. It was Thanksgiving. Everyone was enjoying chicken and dressing, yes, with a side order of ham. Everyone ate except me. The only thing I could consume was one red, cold Popsicle. Yet my body couldn't even keep that inside."

"Greta Long", the nurse called.

I heard it, but I couldn't even walk. So my sister got up first and took hold of my hand. I managed to creep into the room for the examination.

"So what seems to be the problem?" the doctor asked after he finally came into the cold room.

"My stomach is hurting! I have not had anything to eat in three days!" I told him everything.

Suddenly he looked as if he had seen a ghost. Then he murmured, "We will have to admit you to the hospital immediately."

"Lord how can this be happening? It's only been six weeks since my first surgery! I can't. I can't go through this again!"

I literally crawled from the doctor's office to Mary's car, then from the car to the emergency room. The receptionist in the hospital quickly found me a room, and explained that the doctor requested that a feeding tube be ordered for me.

"Please help me somebody. I am hungry, but nothing will stay on my stomach".

I lay in the bed with tears in my eyes hoping that everything would be all right.

"Maybe after this surgery they will find out why my body is rejecting nourishment. I hope my release date will be before Christmas because that blue shimmering pantsuit will look great on my thinning body. That was my ultimate goal."

"I was tired of being referred to as 'fat' and 'chubby'. So I bought the pantsuit to give me courage to go through with my first weight-loss surgery.

"Oh goodness, my surgery is scheduled for tomorrow."

"Oh, God, something is truly wrong! I can not even walk upright."

"The pain keeps hitting my already mangled body. Can I take this torture again and survive?"

I asked my sister to get my life insurance policy out of the basement. The policy explained that Mary would be the executor of my estate at the time of my death.

I lay in the hospital bed agonizing. I was only 50 years old, but I felt as if my time was running out.

"I tossed and turned all night praying because I am scared," I told Mary.

When I did wake up the next morning I said, "Finally, I can see the sun shinning through the half-opened curtains. The smell of bacon and eggs are coming from the patient's tray in the bed next to me."

"I am so hungry!" I cried as the tears welled up inside and started to trickle down my cheeks.

"I know I can't eat because I have a feeding tube in my weak, despondent body. "

Finally the nurse came in to take me to the operating room in spite of my being sad and angry.

"If you would like a few minutes before we carry her up, you may," the nurse told my children and family members who had begun to arrive.

"They shouldn't cry," I thought as they started a family prayer. "You shouldn't kiss my tear-stained face. You act as if I'm not coming back!"

"I can hardly speak because the attendant has drugged me and I am drifting off to sleep."

"Oh no. Oh no. I can see my body lying on the table? What do you mean that my blood pressure is dropping?"

"Oh no! No!" They pronounced me dead at 11:00 A.M.

I died trying to become thin
Not realizing beauty comes from within.
On a quest to become what some thought I should be –
Forgetting God had a unique plan for me.
Now I am dead and my breath has ceased.
Remember to love yourself for who you are.
God made you a special shining star.
Bye,

Greta Long

Footnote: "Since Stephanie (who is the author of this book) and I had the same problems, she will finish speaking for me and others who died due to the complications of weight loss surgery. Please listen to her. Remember that surgery to improve your appearance is meaningless if you do not love yourself beforehand. I wished someone would have warned me."

What is Weight-Loss Surgery?

Greta Long, an acquaintance that I met only once, had a dying request that her sister Mary shared with me. That dying request was for me to plead with others to get all of the details about weight loss-surgery before agreeing to be a victim as she and I were. Read first my ordeal.

Let's begin by discussing weight loss surgery for severe obesity. Obesity is defined as a chronic condition that is very difficult to treat. Yet surgery to promote weight loss by restricting food intake or interrupting digestive processes is said to be an option for severely obese people.

In technical terms, a body mass index above 40, which means about 100 pounds overweight for men and about 80 pounds for women, indicates that a person is severely obese and therefore a candidate for surgery.

I learned that the concept of weight loss surgery grew out of the results of operations - some for cancer and some for severe ulcers where there is a removal of large portions of the stomach or the small intestine. Study has shown that at first, patients undergoing this procedure tended to lose weight rapidly after surgery. So some physicians began to use such an operation to treat severe obesity. The first operation that was widely used was the intestinal by-pass. The operation that was first used 40 years ago produced weight-loss by causing mal-absorbing.

The original idea was that patients could eat large amounts of food, which would be poorly digested or passed along too fast for the body to absorb many calories.

Surgeons now use techniques that produce weight loss primarily by limiting how much the stomach can hold. Many stomachs can only hold up to two ounces of food at a time.

From my study, I came to the realization that some doctors pressure many obese people into weight-loss surgery. The patients are told that it is their "last chance" and without it they "will certainly die" of weight complications. Many doctors believe that a certain set of complications can be attributed to high weight gain alone. Unfortunately, this piece of knowledge has never been proven by respectable research.

Obnoxiously some obese people are rejected by their doctors and refused any further treatment unless they agree to undergo the surgery. Patients are told that the procedures have been improved in recent years and are better than ever. Patients are told how "easy" it will be to lose weight after the surgery and how much better their lives will be when they are thinner.

The truth is that while fewer people today

die on the operation table or from a direct result of the surgery, many still die earlier than their projected life span. Many others die later of factors less directly related to the surgery, but deaths are brought on by complications from it anyway. Most who survive do so with a severely compromised quality of life, a greatly shortened life span and sometimes no great weight loss in the long run.

The most important factor about weight-loss surgery is the risk. This part is close to my soul because I experienced so many complications. I have had to be hospitalized over twenty-six times. This has simply made me realize that the negative side effects have taken over my life.

First, there is the emotional distress because of the small food intake that the body can hold. This was my greatest obstacle. I really feared losing my mind. I was hungry. I could only eat small portions of unfulfilling foods.

Other common effects include serious vitamin and mineral deficiencies of the body. There are also drastic results of anemia, hair loss, chronic dehydration and vomiting. I experienced all of these life hindrances. Oh how I regret having weight-loss surgery. Directly I experienced, after surgery, ripped stitches and staples in the stomach wall.

There is a possibility that a patient can sometimes suffer from contamination of the abdominal cavity from leakage. There may be a problem of devices that don't work properly or devices that come loose, devices that block the intestinal tract, and degradation of stomach tissue that is confined and unused.

The effects of such drastic contusions to the body and restriction to its basic functions are numerous and can take many forms. Because of this, we may never know how many survivors of weight-loss surgery died of its complications, directly or indirectly because the effects worsened or other medical conditions of the body developed.

It is sad that many people are not happy with themselves because society has instilled in us that we are to be "thin to fit in". Daily images of the "perfect body" are plastered on videos and magazines. Then people who are overweight are enticed to try anything to become thin. Unfortunately, if you are overweight, the world sometimes looks past you.

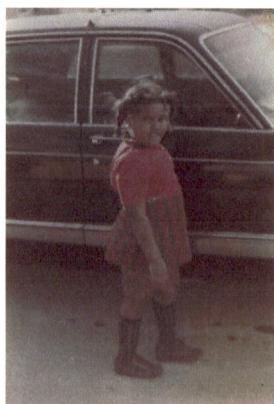

Age 5 (150 pounds)

My Personal Battle

It is strange that a person can be invisible at 370 pounds. Most people never really looked me in my big, brown eyes to see the real Stephanie. Maybe this is the reason I almost "died trying to become thin". I thought that losing weight would be my key to fitting into society. I now realize that if you do not love yourself before the weight is off, it is almost impossible to love yourself when the process is finished.

I took drastic measures to become thin. If only I had exercised the faith in God that I always talked about, maybe continual suffering would not have become a part of my life.

I can't speak for everyone but Gastric bypass surgery for obese conditions was one of the worst decisions I could have made.

If you are considering this surgery, please pray, if you believe in prayer. At least research the positive and the negative side effects. Most of all, remember that this is a process in which your family and friends will also be affected. My very presence on this earth, at this moment is only by the grace of God because with all of my complications, I should be dead. In fact, sit back and fasten your seatbelt as I take you on a roller coaster ride through the doors of death that I faced.

Interestingly, God spoke the same words to

Satan about me as He did about His servant Job.

She belongs to me
And the Lord said to Satan,
Behold, she is in thine hand but save her life
(Reference – JOB 3:6)

All of my life I had been overweight. In fact, in first grade I weighed 150 pounds. At that stage, other children were very cruel. They called me "pig" and "fatty". But in spite of this, I always had dreams that one day I would be smaller.

The teachers didn't help the situation either. In second grade they "chose" me to play Santa Claus in the Christmas play. I was so happy at first, but later I realized that the part was not because of my talent. I had been selected because I "looked like Saint Nick."

I cried. After all, as a child this was humiliating.

I tried a variety of other weight loss methods but if they did not quickly start to work in a couple of months I gave up trying the techniques. I thought that "Weight-Loss Surgery" was my only way out. Then people would stop talking about me. However this procedure opened up a bigger, festered sore that took so much time to heal.

Oh sure I would have the latest fashions, and shine like the colors of a big beautiful rainbow, so I thought. I dreamed that men would also be knocking at my door every day asking me out on dates. This was a lie from the pit of hell. The devil had plans to destroy me physically and spiritually, because of my fleshly desires.

> *St. John 10:10 – The thief cometh not, but*
> *for to steal, and to kill, and to destroy:*
> *I am come that they might have life, and that*
> *They might have it more abundantly.*

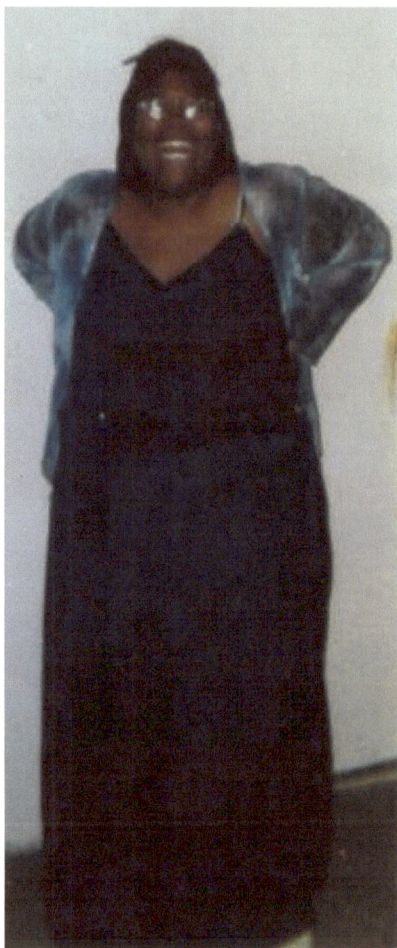

290 pounds (at home in Mississippi)
1999 before surgery

Why Wait?

Believe it or not, I had a one-sided conversation with God, even after I had read brochures about the surgery. I said, *"Lord I can't wait on you. I want this weight gone right now. It is taking too long for you to help me. Please let me do this my way. I want a husband and I am going to get him when I lose weight."* You see, at that time I was dating someone, but he had not asked me to marry him.

When I finally made up my mind, (God didn't say anything). I felt as if I was Cinderella at the ball as the clock struck midnight because a desired reality was about to become visible.

Yes, to wait on God is to trust in His word. I did not wait because we did not have a strong relationship. I was focusing on "me", "myself", and "I", which was selfish thinking. God's plan for my life never did manifest itself before there was total submission to Him.

My thinking was so messed up because I felt that my slobbish, fat, dependent days were over, and then a thin, trimmed, and independent woman had evolved in my flesh. Weight Loss surgery would be my way out of a lifetime of misery. Little did I know that my train ride to spiritual and physical suicide was only about to begin. Waiting on the Lord was hard for me because I felt as if life was passing by me.   I know now that there is a reward for waiting on the LORD.

God's Plan

ISAIAH 40:31

They that wait upon the Lord shall renew their strength;
They shall mount up with wings as eagles;
they shall run, and not be weary;
and they shall walk, and not faint

My focus was on temporary pleasures in this life and not on my eternal crown. This was wrongful thinking because I knew that as a Christian we should be preparing to spend eternity with God.

So, I say to you, people, please consult God when you are making any decisions. He will let us know the direction in which to go. My mind was already made up and nobody or nothing was going to interfere in my life-changing decision - not even God.

PROVERBS 3:5-6

5) **Trust in the Lord with all thine heart and lean not unto thine own understanding.**
6) **In all thy ways acknowledge Him, and He shall direct thy paths.**

Yes, God was aware of my motives. Yes, He allowed his permissible will to be done in my life because of my disobedience. Think about it, I'm the one who told God what I was going to do. At that time, I could not tell you why I should have desired something so bad that I would go against God's wishes!

Rebellion will cause God to stand back and let you have what you think is best. Just remember that our Father does know what is best. The real reason I was so anxious is because lust had taken over me. I thought losing weight would make a certain young man that I had been dating, marry me. Now I know that if someone loves you they will accept you for what and who you are and for how you actually look. I am not blaming him for my misfortunes because I realize that I had major issues before I met the young man that I liked.

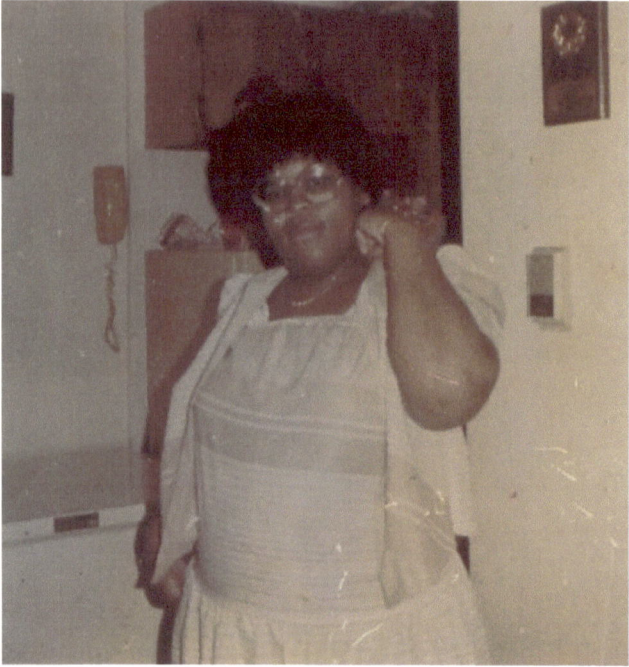

290 pounds, at home in Mississippi

The Decision

How did I arrive at this point?

I was sitting one day and I began to think of how it would feel to be two dress sizes smaller. I need for you to understand that most of my life people have treated me differently because of my weight.

I did not have a prom date. I was not asked out to parties while in high school. Many nights I cried myself to sleep praying that God would just spare me from pain. I even tried to commit suicide because of my weight.

Then finally I made the decision to undergo surgery. I went to the doctor's office to see if I was a good candidate. In other words, to be eligible for surgery a person needed a body mass index above 40-percent, which means about 100 pounds overweight for men and about 80 pounds for women. Sure, I no doubt would qualify, because my weight had ballooned to 320 pounds. Therefore after my examination the doctor said the magic words, "YES". I fit the weight profile.

I left the doctor's office and went home excited. The only things pending were the approval from my insurance company and a psychological evaluation to see if I was emotionally strong enough. I had no doubts about that.

I had done my own research. I also called a

lady who I heard had undergone weight-loss surgery earlier. She told me, as I am telling you, "to research the procedure". She pointed out her good-looking figure and her new hairstyle, and the fact that she was still alive. Then later I found out that she forgot to mention the blood clots that she had incurred **after** surgery. Since she didn't mention it, never once did I look for information and research the dangerous side effects. My mind was set and no matter what anybody said, including God, I was not going to turn back.

In my mind, the entrapped caterpillar was about to emerge into a big, beautiful butterfly. Did I pray? Yes, I said self-centered prayers, but the decision was already made.

I was so excited that I did not stop to think that the enemy was sitting back laughing at me because through my disobedience to God a door had been left open in which he could come. What the heck, my fellowship with God was already broken. I had started to participate in sinful activities and it did not even bother me. The insurance company gave the final approval for me after a month. However, at first, I did not pass my psychological evaluation. The tests revealed that I was not emotionally strong enough to handle the emotional stress that comes after surgery.

I believe that even the day before surgery, that God was trying to get my attention, but I went to a psychiatrist instead.

A psychiatrist approved me for surgery!

At least, I humbled myself enough to approach my pastor and I told him about the surgery. At first, he just listened. However, a few days later he said that the Lord spoke to him and told him to tell me that I should not have the surgery. My decision was made though. Yes, God was trying to help me. God unfortunately, even knew what I was about to face. He only wanted to save me from the misery.

My mother was also very concerned. After talking with some people on her job, she found out that even her supervisor at work had the same type of surgery. The supervisor told her that after 10 years she was still severely sick sometimes. In fact, she gained all of her weight back.

Did that information make a difference? I still did not care what anybody said. This surgery and new body would be my dream come true.

My church family prayed for me but this did not change my decision. I was acting like Jonah when he was told to go to Nineveh and preach. Instead he went to Tar'shish. Therefore believe it or not, I paid the price just as Jonah did.

The Day of Surgery

I woke up the morning of March 14, 2000 and laid in my bed thinking,

"After today my life will never be the same again."

Go ahead and laugh now. See, I could not eat breakfast before surgery, nor eat anything after midnight. I got up, prayed, and took my bath. I thought about canceling but it was only a few hours away and I was tired of being fat. The surgery was scheduled for 11:00 A.M. but I had to be there by 7:30 A.M. So my Aunt Gloria and I caught the bus to the hospital. When we arrived, I was quickly admitted. They took me to a room and started administering an I.V (intravenous tube of liquid). I still kept defending myself.

Some of you know that society can be so cruel to those who are overweight. I know this sounds stupid to others but until you have "walked a mile in my shoes," please don't try to judge me. Just read Greta Long's story again, and then read my story. After that, try to imagine what you probably would do.

I was so scared. Then I prayed again as the anesthesiologist came in and talked to me. Next he gave me a sedative. The attendant took me in a room and that is the last thing I remember until about 7:00 P.M. when I became strongly conscious. As soon as my eyes opened I quickly regretted my decision. The pain was so bad. I was hooked up to all types of equipment. I had and I.V. in my arm and neck, and another one (called a cathartic instrument) to help me use the bathroom because I could not get out of bed. The morphine was so strong and all I could say then was "Lord I am sorry."

I was hungry but I could only intake ice chips. Even this made me so hungry. I stayed in the intensive care room for 2 days with no food. I had to wear an oxygen mask to help me breathe. I suddenly realized that this was a serious surgery. Reality had just set in.

When they moved me into a regular room I had staples in my stomach and a tube also to drain the fluid out of my stomach. I could not digest anything but liquids. I was painfully hungry and distressed. I began wishing that I could turn back the clock hands.

From then on, I was always in constant pain. One time I did not have a bowel movement for seven days. My face had big, dime-sized spots everywhere. I was suffering so much because of my disobedience to God.

What was strange though was that my doctor said he could not find any physical reason why I was having so many problems. Therefore he said it must have been all in my mind. This comment hurt me really bad because I knew how my body was feeling.

Going Home

Saturday, March 18, 2000 was my discharge date. Aunt Gloria and my cousin Angela came to get me. I was so hungry when I got home I could not lay down straight. Would you believe my Aunt cooked chicken that night? The smell and sight of the food upset me because I could dissolve only liquids. Oh God, I was so hungry. My diet consisted of liquids and pureed food for 4 weeks. The devil began to joyfully attack me because my mind was not on the Lord. My mind was on my circumstances.

I realized then that any time you take your eyes off the Lord you are in trouble.

For the first two weeks, everything was fine. However, around the third week the depression set in. I could not focus on anything because of my small consumption of food. I could only eat about 1 ounce of food at a time. I had to go to a doctor who prescribed me an antidepressant drug. This medicine made me sick because I was not supposed to have any solid pills until about 3 months later. I felt sick and disoriented. I walked around the house like a zombie.

My body was so out-of-sync that having a bowel movement on my own was void. Therefore, I had to take laxatives almost every day. My first hospital visit was 6 weeks after surgery because my stomach was hurting. As a matter of fact that very day the pain was so intense that I could hear the devil saying, "Cut your stomach open. Then your pain will leave." I remembered that I had gotten the scissors and placed them at the top of the scar on my mangled stomach when God spoke.

He said, "You can't kill yourself because you belong to Me and you did not give yourself life."

---

2 CORINTHIANS 5:7

We live by what we believe, not by what we see.

Immediately I dropped the big, black scissors and began to sob uncontrollably. Again, I realized that any time you take your eyes off the Lord you are in trouble.

Even after that ordeal, I needed to have a second surgery 5 months later. The doctors had to remove my gall bladder because I had gallstones. This made me even more depressed. The chaplain in the hospital visited me and said, "If you feel like you are at the end of your rope, tie a knot and hang on." I took her advice and began to praise God for my healing even though I was severely hurting.

I was always in constant pain.

ISAIAH 53:5
But he was wounded
for the wrong we did;
He was crushed
for the evil we did.
The punishment,
which made us well,
was given to him,
and we are healed
because of his wounds.

Pages From My Diary
(Unedited Version)

March 13 2000
This is the month for my surgery. I am very excited and scared. The date for surgery is March 14, 11:30 A.M. The psyche (psychological) evaluation did not go well. I had to get a second opinion to see if I will be a good candidate. Didn't find out for sure that the surgery was on until March 13 at 2:00 p.m. I am so glad but was worried about complications.

March 14 2000
I woke up early feeling good knowing in a couple of hours my life will change forever. Made it to the hospital with my aunt by my side. I was very nervous when they called my name. It was hard for them to find a vein. The nurse had to stick me several times.

They wheeled me to the waiting room and gave me medicine through my I.V. to relax me. I couldn't breathe. I didn't complain. I began to pray. The nurse finally took me in the surgery room and moved me to another bed. That is all I remember. I woke up around 7:00 P.M. feeling crazy. Lord I was hurting so badly. I didn't cry but prayed. Thank God, for his word it helped me so much

March 15 2000
Still hurting. Slept most of the day when the nurses weren't sticking and pulling on me. I am still hurting very much. The morphine helped a lot. I really regret having this surgery. Lord what was I thinking? However, it is too late to turn back the hands of time.

March 16 2000

Had juice and a Popsicle but I want some real food. maybe I can sneak me some. Removed catheter and one I.V. made me get up and wash up so I could move out of intensive care. feel better. prayer helps. My Aunt and cousin visited that evening. I walked by myself today.

March 17 2000

Eating a little. going to bathroom by myself. My friend Barry visited. Pastor Orlando and Yvonne Lewis visited me. they brought me a pretty flower and balloon. Aunt and cousin visited. My mom called. today is her birthday. Doctor said I can go home tomorrow. Took 2 tubes out of my stomach.

March 18 2000

Finally going home. moving a little better. I am so hungry.

April 3 2000 (last entry)

I am feeling down and lonely but God is here with me. I have lost 17.5 pounds thank God. Feel a little better. Need to get out of this house. My car is breaking down. I feel kind of uncomfortable. Have to keep my focus on Jesus and hold on to his hand. Depression is trying to take over. Lord Please Help Me.

The Results

Yes, I lost 100 pounds in only four months. Then my body went into shock. I could barely walk. I would always stay in the bed for three, or four days, barely able to get up. Nor was I even able to use the bathroom, or brush my teeth. My family and some of my friends were there for me. However, I found out who really cared about me when I was sick.

I had to stop attending college for one year and had to return to my hometown so that someone could care for me.

One day when I could feel myself dying, I lay in the bed and said, "God, if it is my time to leave I am ready."

But guess what? My body began to function again. Yes there were some positive outcomes, but the negatives outweighed the positives. Positively, I lost a total of 120 pounds. My weight dropped from a size 26-28. I could then wear clothing sizes 14-16. Yet today however I still have excess skin on my body and I do not have the money to have it removed. On television, when stars have this surgery, they have the money to have other surgeries if needed but this is unfortunate for others in my case.

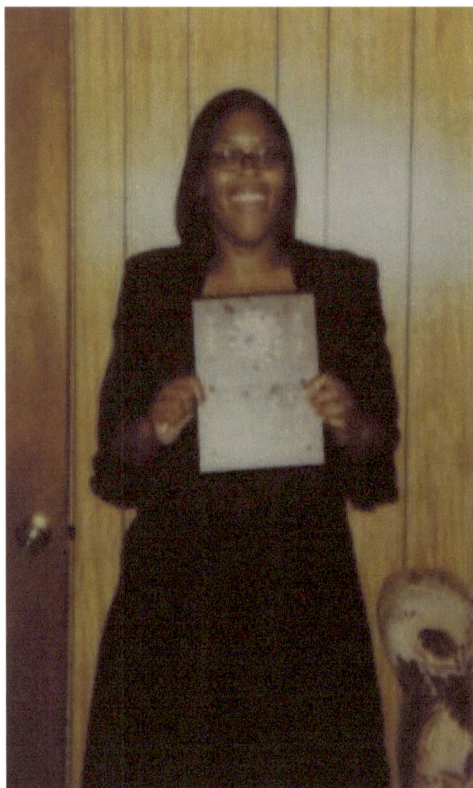

Stephanie in 2003; 3 years after the surgery
Don't let the smile deceive you.

The Complications

I was sick for approximately two years. Many days the pain was so unbearable I did not sleep peacefully. Sometimes I needed to have help getting out of the bathtub and going to the bathroom. I would grind my teeth together because the pain was constant and painful. It felt as if someone was kicking me in the stomach with a hard boot. The pain never stopped.

"Can I survive these terrible days?" I would ask myself.

Have you ever heard someone screaming in your mind and in reality, it's really your voice. On my most dreadful days, I would ask God to let me die because my strength was no longer sufficient. The spark that once filled my eyes had turned to darkness. It's awful when you can't die, but you have no desire to live.

Isaiah 40: 31

They that wait upon the Lord
shall renew their strength;
They shall mount up
with wings as eagles;
They shall run,
and not be weary;
And they shall walk,
and not faint.

Life After Death

I am so glad that GOD kept me alive because my story will help other people realize that weight-loss surgery is not a magical solution.

There is a lot at stake. Even after surgery, some people do gain weight back. One doctor told me that after about 2 years the stomach begins to expand again.

Come to think of it, I know a lady who gained all of the weight back after about 10 years. I have gained some weight and it's only been about 4 years since my surgery.

This is heartbreaking because of the entire trauma I go through. If only people could love themselves the way God loves us, this would be so awesome.

I am sitting here realizing God's love for me is unconditional and this is the way He wants us to love others. We all are unique individuals born into this world for his purpose

---

REVELATION 4:9
Thou art worthy, O Lord, to receive glory and honour and power: for thou hast
created all things, and for thy pleasure they are and were created.

Through all of the obstacles of weight loss surgery God has made me stronger and more compassionate. There was a time when I did not have compassion. So many Christians want to do their own thing; therefore they end up on the sidelines of the race wounded, weary, and sad.

God is my source of strength now. Trying to be what others wanted me to be made me search for happiness in *things* instead of finding comfort in the God who made all things. God is my provider. Please, let God shape and mold you into what he has predestined you to be. Trust in God; not man, for your needs.

JEREMIAH 17:5-8

5 This is what the LORD says: "A curse is
placed on those who trust other people.
who depend on humans for strength,
who have stopped trusting the LORD.
6 They are like a bush in a desert
that grows in a land where no one lives,
a hot and dry land with bad soil.
They don't know about the good things
God can give.
7 But the person who trusts in the LORD
will be blessed. The LORD will show
him that He can be trusted.
8 He will be strong, like a tree planted near
water that sends its roots by a stream.
It is not afraid when the days are hot;
its leaves are always green.
It does not worry in a year when no rain
comes; it always produces fruit.

God is the potter and we are the clay. God is
on the potter's wheel shaping us into purpose. Some
people are fighting against his purpose. The Lord
wants you to be a plate, but in the flesh, you are
trying to work against Him and be a cup. I am
learning to be obedient to my LORD because I have
experienced first hand what disobedience can bring
to a person.

> ... as the clay is in the potter's hand, so are ye in mine hand, O house of Israel.
> Jeremiah 18:6

REBELLION

Just as with Jonah, God said, "Wait". My response was, "I am going to have this surgery, Lord, no matter what you say".

Now, I am telling anyone who is reading this book, "Do not rebel against God because He loves you. If He says 'no' or 'wait', there is a reason. God knows the plans He has for us."

Jennie's Decision

After all, that I have been through, God has instructed me to tell my testimony to whomever He sends in my direction. There are many times that I have had conversations about my surgery moreover, someone will say, "I know someone who is thinking about the procedure." Or the person speaking states that they want to have it performed for himself or herself.

In fact, one day a lady named Jennie was talking to me about having the surgery. I told her to pray and research the procedure. I shared my story with her to let her know that the decision affects everyone who loves her. She listened to me and decided not to have the surgery.

Another Day

I often reminisce about being in the hospital:

Now that I lay here meditating on what I have done, I wonder do the other patients, who will come through this mess, fully comprehend what I am saying about the procedure. In fact, now that I'm writing this book I go back over what I was told by the doctor. I need to know, "Did I understand that dribble?"

Well readers, you are so intelligent. Yet a sickening feeling down in my stomach is hunching me saying, "Stephanie, let them know what the operational preparation material said. Then if they can fully understand and still want to take this drastic step through pain and agony, at least you have warned them." So here we go, back through the time tunnel.

Getting My Consent for the Gastric Bypass Surgery

I knew I wanted the gastric bypass surgery. However, I did not know all of the processes involved that are needed to have a successful surgery.

The doctor explained that Gastric bypass for obesity would be an operation to create a small food pouch at the upper end of my stomach disabling me so that I would only have a capacity of less than two ounces. The pouch is connected to the upper small outlet of about 1.0 cm in diameter, or just say ½ inch. By "bypassing" the remaining portion of the stomach, you get the technical term Gastric Bypass. This would limit the amount of food or liquid I could eat or drink at one time. Since my intake would be restricted, if I would consume too much at one meal, I would begin to feel full and would even vomit until I learned how much my stomach would hold.

Following the operation, I became intolerant of refined sugars, which caused unpleasant symptoms of nausea, shaking, sweating, and even weakness. This always lasted from a few minutes to a half-hour. This side effect (dumping) was particularly useful in reinforcing good dietary habits and helping me maintain weight loss on a long term. However, I must stay away from sweets to avoid the aforementioned symptoms.

Is it possible to "beat the system"? I read that by continuously drinking high calorie liquids throughout the day a person can fail to lose weight. However, if I ate a balanced diet at normal meal times, my caloric intake would be reduced and I would definitely lose more weight.

The brochures that I read stated that most patients lose about one third of their starting weight at a rate of approximately 10 pounds per month over the 9 to 15 months after surgery. Weight loss then would level off and even stabilize at an average of 30% above the standard weight for height, as determined by the Metropolitan Life Tables, 1983.

Please readers, please remember that surgery for obesity involves major surgery and has risks and potential complications. You must be aware of these complications before your operation. The research will tell you that as with all surgery, complications include heart and lung problems, bleeding, infection, and blood clots in the legs and lungs. These complications are all more common among obese patients. There are other complications specifically related to gastric bypass. I found out that peptic ulcers occur in about 2% of patients after surgery, and because the spleen lies close to the upper end of the stomach where the surgery is performed, injury to the spleen is possible and removal of the spleen may be necessary. This is an infrequent occurrence; however, it's happening in less than 1% of patients. In about the same number of cases though, perforation of the stomach, or leak at the staple line or hood up between stomach and upper small intestine with leakage of stomach contents may occur within the first few days after surgery. This serious complication requires immediate re-operation to close the perforation or leak.

Also, one cause of this life-threatening complication is failure of the patient to comply with fluid and dietary restriction instructions after surgery. Injury to the vagus nerves to the stomach is a possibility. Since these nerves control the rate of stomach emptying, this may result in delayed emptying of the stomach. Again, these complications are stated to be uncommon.

With long-term follow-up after this type of surgery, an increasing number of staple-line failures have been reported, rising as high as 15% or more after 10 years. Surgical re-stapling is then required. To prevent this, the stomach is no longer simply proportioned with a row of staples, but is now completely divided between two rows of staples, using the technique known as "Transected Gastric Bypass". Staple-line failure is uncommon with this technique. The two parts of the stomach can be reconnected in the future, should this ever be required, although weight gain would then recur.

The mortality rate of gastric bypass is less than 1%, but both you and your family members should realize that gastric bypass is major surgery and that complication of this procedure can be fatal. Are you willing to take the chance?

Of all these factors, there could also be no guarantee of weight-loss success. There were many alternatives in the management of obesity, particularly various dietary regimes that carry their own potential risk of complications. Yet I had the surgery though because I believed surgical treatment was a management alternative and I did consider it as such. Unfortunately, it was not an absolute cure-all and it tremendously did not have an effect on the underlying causes of my obesity. I realize now that the underlying causes were psychologically, physically motivated, environmentally motivated, due to familiar surroundings and was hormonal. In most ways, I guess surgery was successful in achieving some weight loss.

PATIENT SELECTION

I can't keep from emphasizing that the gastric bypass surgeries are major operations with short and long-term complications. Some of the complications remain to be completely elucidated. Unfortunately, there are insufficient data on which to base sound recommendations for patient selection using objective clinical parameters alone. However, from other readings from the material that the doctor gave me the study showed that while data accumulates, it might be possible in certain cases to consider surgery on the bases of limited information from the uncontrolled or short-term follow-up studies available. This will involve an assessment of the risk-benefit ratio in each individual case.

As I did, patients should have a complete medical evaluation by a multidisciplinary team with experience in obesity management. You must discuss all treatment options. I was told that only those patients judged by experienced clinicians, to have a low probability of success with non-surgical measures as demonstrated by previous failures in established weight control programs or substantial reluctance to enter such a program, should be considered for surgery.

> A gastric restrictive or bypass procedure should only be considered for well-informed and motivated adult patients with acceptable operative risks. The patient should have the capacity to ensure participation in treatment for a long-term follow-up.

Patients whose BMI exceeds 40 may be considered for surgery if they strongly desire substantial weight loss because obesity severely impairs the quality of their lives. Patients must clearly demonstrate realistic understanding of how you and your family's lives may change after the operation.

I had a significant interference with my lifestyle (e.g. body size problems precluding or severely interfering with employment, family functions, etc.). Sometimes I hurt so badly that I could not stand up straight enough to go to work.

Even now, I have nightmares just thinking about what I went through. I more often remember A GASTROSTOMY TUBE that was placed in the main portion of my stomach during surgery.

The tube acted as a safety valve against the possibility of blockage occurring at the small bowel hook-up. This was done so that there would be no complication of secretions. The secretion would come from my stomach, pancreas, and upper small intestine. The secretion would also come from my bile, or from the liver that may have become trapped in the segment closed above by the new staple line and below by the postoperative blockage.

I was told that this usually would be due to swelling, bleeding, adhesions, or kinking at the new hook-up. As a routine, the tube drained into a bag for 3 days after surgery, and then it was plugged off. It was removed at the first office visit when the staples were to be removed. Your doctor should definitely explain additional risks and alternatives. Be sure to ask many questions.

Just think. In Greta Long's case so voluminous were the secretions that the stomach and intestine distended rapidly, and the patient, Greta Long went into shock, requiring another, immediate operation. Remember Greta Long? She died.

Greta Long went into shock. Another immediate operation was required. Yes, remember Greta Long? She died!

If you don't have personal relationships with God, say this prayer and start to live.

Prayer for Salvation

Father,

You loved the world so much, you gave your only begotten son to die for our sins so that whoever believes in him will not perish, but have eternal life. God, your word says that we are saved by grace through faith as a gift from you. There is nothing we can do to earn salvation.

I believe and confess with my mouth that Jesus Christ is your son, the Savior of the world. I believe that he died on the cross for me, and bore all of my sins - paying the price for me. I believe in my heart that you raised Jesus from the dead.

I ask you to forgive my sins. I confess Jesus as my Lord according to your word. I am saved and will spend eternity with you!
Thank you, Father. I am so grateful.

In Jesus name,
Amen

Read
John 3:16   _Ephesians 2:8, 9_
Romans 10: 9,10   _I Corinthians 15:3, 4_
     I John 1:9; 4:14-16; 5:1, 12, 13

"GOD LOVES YOU"

God loves you
No matter what you have done
He gave Jesus, His only Son

God loves you
There's eternal life in His name
Acknowledge Him first in all your ways

God loves you
We were made in His image
And the work He has begun in you
He promises to finish

God loves you
Continue to give Him your best
Let Him take control of your life
He will do the rest

by *Stephanie French*
From her first book *SPIRITUAL EMOTIONS*

"STORM"

Trouble and pain tried to control my life
Storm, you can't destroy me
I am safe in my Father's arms

The tears told me they would overtake my spirit
No, they won't
I can call on God, the keeper of my soul

Storm you can't destroy me
I am standing on solid ground

A voice whispered into my ear
that unbelief would kidnap me
This will not stand
I am holding to God's hand

Storm you don't have authority over me
In Jesus' name
Move storm, move

by Stephanie French
From her first book, *SPIRITUAL EMOTIONS*

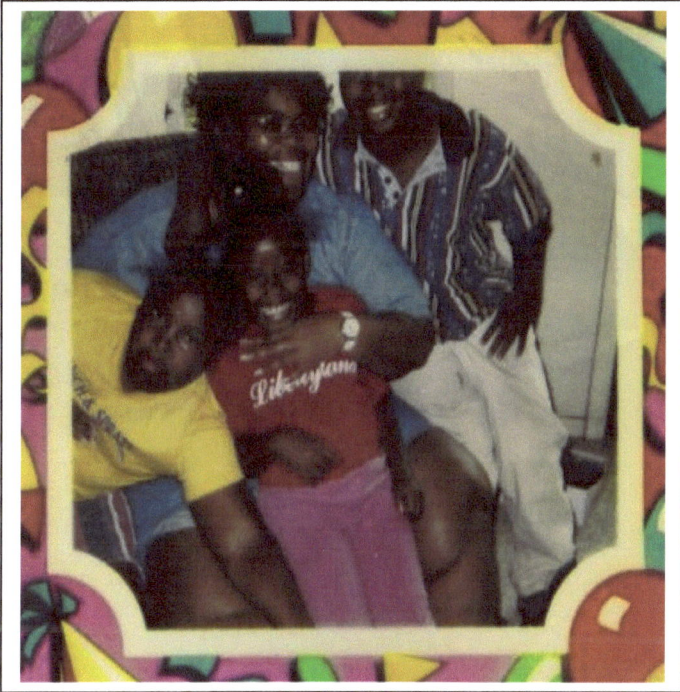

Stephanie (center) and children (l-r): Ashley,
Amber, and DeMario

Oh house of Israel can not I
do with you as this potter?
saith the Lord,
Behold, as the clay is in the
potter's hand
So are ye in mine hand
O house of Israel

"The Potter and Clay"
Jeremiah 18:6

God's Plan
Jeremiah 29:11

For I know the thoughts that I think
towards you,
saith the Lord,
Thoughts of peace, and not of evil,
To give you an expected end.

Glossary

According to research, a number of operations have been performed and discarded as inefficacious or have been discarded because of patient complications. Two operational procedures dominated the medical practice in the early 1990's:

Vertical banded gastro-plastic – a small (10-15-cc) pouch with a restricted outlet along the lesser curvature of the stomach so that the pouch is externally reinforced to prevent disruption or dilation.

Gastric bypass – construction of a proximal gastric pouch whose outlet is a "Y-shaped" limb of a small bowel in varying lengths.

Biliary-pancreatic bypass – a diversion of bile and pancreatic juice that passes into the distal ileum and has a gastric restriction

Sponsor

Gloria Marshall,
Seamstress
-Perfect Stitch-
For additional information contact
(314) 869-4305

M.O.R.E. Publishers Corp.

©2006

54

www.ingramcontent.com/pod-product-compliance
Lightning Source LLC
Chambersburg PA
CBHW041218270326
41931CB00001B/23